YOUR KNOWLEDGE HAS VALUE

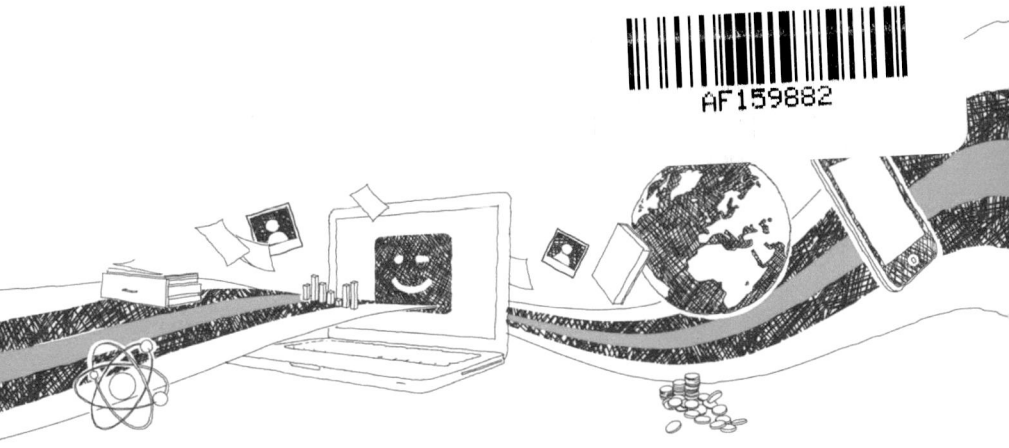

- We will publish your bachelor's and master's thesis, essays and papers

- Your own eBook and book - sold worldwide in all relevant shops

- Earn money with each sale

Upload your text at www.GRIN.com
and publish for free

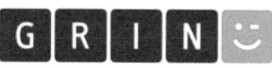

Bibliographic information published by the German National Library:

The German National Library lists this publication in the National Bibliography; detailed bibliographic data are available on the Internet at http://dnb.dnb.de .

This book is copyright material and must not be copied, reproduced, transferred, distributed, leased, licensed or publicly performed or used in any way except as specifically permitted in writing by the publishers, as allowed under the terms and conditions under which it was purchased or as strictly permitted by applicable copyright law. Any unauthorized distribution or use of this text may be a direct infringement of the author s and publisher s rights and those responsible may be liable in law accordingly.

Imprint:

Copyright © 2018 GRIN Verlag
Print and binding: Books on Demand GmbH, Norderstedt Germany
ISBN: 9783668745087

This book at GRIN:

https://www.grin.com/document/428627

Leonard Kahungu

Change Management for Quality Improvement. A Case Study of the Mid Staffordshire Hospital Scandal

GRIN Verlag

GRIN - Your knowledge has value

Since its foundation in 1998, GRIN has specialized in publishing academic texts by students, college teachers and other academics as e-book and printed book. The website www.grin.com is an ideal platform for presenting term papers, final papers, scientific essays, dissertations and specialist books.

Visit us on the internet:

http://www.grin.com/

http://www.facebook.com/grincom

http://www.twitter.com/grin_com

Content

Introduction 2

The Kotter's Analytical Framework 3

Establish a Sense of Urgency 3

Create a Guiding Coalition 4

Develop a Clear Shared Vision 4

Communicate the Vision 5

Empower People to Act on the Vision 5

Create Short Term Wins 5

Consolidate and Build on the Gains 6

Institutionalise the Change 6

Leadership Approaches for Change Management 6

Justification and Conclusions 9

References List 11

Introduction

Guaranteeing that the National Health Service Organisations and the affiliated human resources deliver high quality and equitable care is one of the major priorities in the contemporary health services (Bottle et al., 2011). Yet, the metrics necessary to evaluate the quality and assurance of the healthcare is a matter subject to continuous debate. In the recent past, the concerns associated with the quality of care has attracted wide-ranging interests, particularly by the Mid Staffordshire Hospital scandal. An inquiry report into the Mid Staffordshire NHS Foundation Trust, the Francis Report, released on February 2013 paints a grim picture of the events that transpired during fermentation of the scandal (Francis, 2013). Unfortunately, these events led to the loss of lives, due to issues which could have been managed or addressed better.

Briefly, the Stafford and Cannock Chase hospitals decided to pursue the Foundation Trust in 2005, which was subsequently granted in 2008. However, abnormally high death rates raised eyebrows from various quarters, triggering the formulation of the taskforce to look into the matter (Dixon-Woods et al., 2013). It is largely believed that the scandal was triggered by the quest of the managers to cut down the operational costs and accomplish the minimum labour requirements in attempts to achieve the foundation status and qualify for the NHS trust funds. This indicates that the scandal was as a result of catastrophic organisational challenges that were triggered by poor change management.

Nonetheless, the Mid Staffordshire Hospital has since undergone significant changes as the concerned authorities strive to restore the efficiency and effectiveness of this facility (Salge and Schäfer, 2015). The events that transpired after the scandal was unearthed presents appropriate platform to understand effective change management for quality improvement. The case is also suitable for evaluating how the process of change management since the Mid Stafford Hospital reforms started in 2013 (Francis, 2013). Apparently, the Mid Staffordshire NHS Foundation Trust was placed under the management of the University of North Midlands NHS Trust. At the centre of the scandal, the Stafford Hospital has also renamed to the County Hospital, Stafford, in attempts to create short term wins for the public along with the management. Notably, the County Hospital, Stafford has extensively taken into consideration radical and drastic changes reconstruct the damage sustained in the wake of the Mid Staffordshire NHS Foundation Trust scandal.

The Kotter's Analytical Framework

According to John P Kotter changes in organisational are inevitable and must be evaluated using an eight-step analytical framework, in attempts to ensure that the transition is managed appropriately and successfully. Analysing the changes that the County Hospital, Stafford has undertaken will provide explicit insights on how the facility in collaboration with NHS and other organs in the UK healthcare system attempted to manage changes attributed to post-scandal management and interventions (Mohammed et al., 2013).

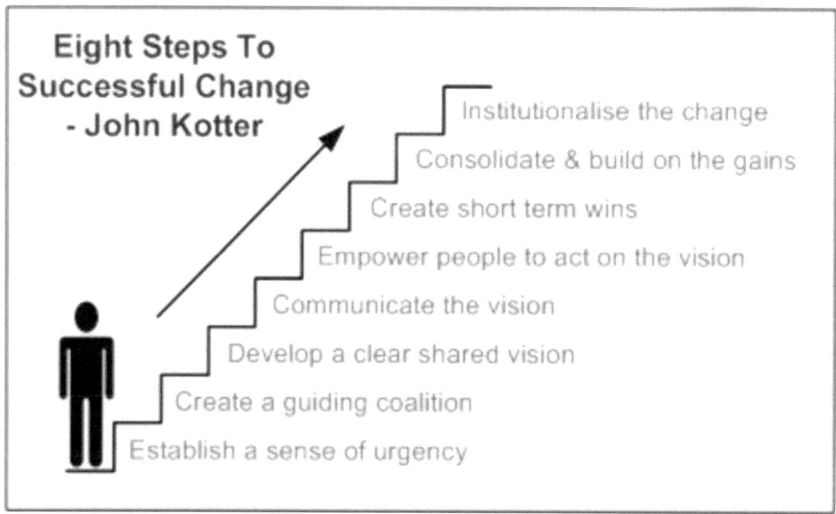

Figure 1 Source (Kotter and Cohen, 2014).

Establish a Sense of Urgency

It is paramount for organisations to be ready and responsive to changes that happen within the organisational environment. According to Kotter, it is imperative to identify potential threats along with the consequences that might emerge in the future when the status quos remains. Evaluating potential opportunities which can be used to establish effective interventions is also paramount (Francis, 2013). This should be followed by the commencement of honest dialogues with the stakeholders. Following the dissolution of the Mid Staffordshire NHS Trust organisation, the management was transferred to the University Hospitals of North Midlands (UHNM) NHS Trust. The UHNM NHS Trust creates a sense of urgency through persistent desires to provide safer services in a conducive environment, in which people get effective treatment along with healthcare services. This is

Create a Guiding Coalition

Kotter observes that change cannot be enforced by a single person alone, but rather a group of people from key positions in different levels of organisation must support the transformation process. The coalition members are required to have leadership, influence, credibility and the necessary expertise in the required change (Traynor, 2014). The UHNM NHS Trust has since partnered with multiple agencies to implement and sustain the change. Some of the notable partnerships are Keele University Faculty of Health along with the Staffordshire University. Most of the medical staffs serving at the County Hospital, Stafford are obtained from the two institutions. This relationship is paramount as it allows the UHNM NHS Trust to consistently ensure that its staffs are trained and guided with respect to the expectations of the local community and also based on the change implementation process (UHNM 2017b). The current hospital staff at the County Hospital, Stafford has also been integrated in the change process in attempts to enhance the outcome in the long run. This coalition is essential in promoting and sustaining change.

Develop a Clear Shared Vision

Managing change requires effective visions and objectives that are explicit and observable to all. The quest to initiate change in the Mid Staffordshire NHS Foundation Trust was based on observable and clear vision, to establish the factors behind increased death rates and poor services in the midst of the inter-organisational and public outcries (Bottle et al., 2011). As previously mentioned, the County Hospital, Stafford is bound to the UHNM NHS Trust management. Thus, this foundation is the primary organisation that is responsible for the development of the facility's vision. In this regards, the UHNM NHS Trust vision states that the primary vision is to become one of the best university teaching hospitals by 2025 in the United Kingdome and subsequently develop a world-class status by the year 2030 (UHNM 2017a). This vision as a guiding principle for constant enhancement of patient care and nurture innovations within the organisation. The UHNM NHS Trust also aspires to provide a safe and attracting working environment for the staff. These visions are essential in influencing the change process within the facility.

Communicate the Vision

Having established the vision, it is paramount to communicate effectively as it provides the guiding principle for initiating change. The UHNM NHS Trust has over five thousand followers on Tweeter and other social network platforms, which allows it to articulate its vision to the public. It has also become vocal in popularising its activities through the main website and affiliate World Wide Web platforms, in which the organisation's vision is explicitly outlined and explained to the public. Besides, the Latest News platform on the UHNM NHS Trust's website constantly communicated with vision (UHNM 2017b). This is essential as it lays a firm foundation to stimulate and manage change within the County Hospital, Stafford.

Empower People to Act on the Vision

Kotter requires the lead change agents to communicate sensible vision to the organisation by removing structural barriers in attempts to make the change proposal compatible with the vision. As a consequence, it is fundamental to provide the required training and align the system with the vision, as well as address resistance from the concerned parties. The staff at the County Hospital has undergone massive and sustained training to enhance the care delivered to the patient. The feedback collection system has also improved as the UHNM NHS Trust engages the public to evaluate and address various issues arising from the treatment. An improved feedback collection mechanism is essential in change management as it empowers all the stakeholders to air their grievances, which reduced possible resistance. It empowers the staff, patients and the general public to keep the management in check to ensure that the vision is delivered according to the expectations (UHNM 2017a).

Create Short Term Wins

The County Hospital has developed a framework, which allows it to acquire monthly quality and safety reports. This allows the public and the staff to assess short term wins due to the change implemented in the organisation. The County Hospital opened two new wards in 2017, a Renal Unit and an Elective Orthopaedic Unit. The resulting expansion allows the staff to have a spacious and developed working environment while the Stafford community can access these services closer home. The new wards allow the patients, their relatives and the staffs permits sufficient rooms for confidential conversations, which are essential in enhancing the quality of the treatment process (UHNM 2017b). An audit by the Trauma Audit and Research Network indicates that for one thousand major trauma clients treated at the UHNM NHS Trust, including the County Hospital, thirteen people survived who would not have survived traumatic incidents. This is one of the major short-term gain observed at the hospital since the transformation process started. Moreover, the County Hospital has quadrupled the number of rooms to increase the capacity and also developed new services such as plastic surgery, eye surgery and orthopaedic surgery. These short term gains are essential in supporting the change process in the facility.

Consolidate and Build on the Gains

More changes are paramount in consolidating the gains obtained during the change initiation process. Constant training of the staff and monthly performance evaluation at the team, division, area, committee and Trust Board levels are some of the strategic approaches that have been taken to consolidate changes at the facility. In particular, performance indicators play a central role in assessing the change management and also evaluating whether the primary objectives and cumulative goals align with the County Hospital's vision (UHNM 2017a).

Institutionalise the Change

Lastly, it is inevitable to institutionalise the change, based on the findings and recommendations developed from the change management process. Constant performance evaluation and management as observed in the consolidation of change allows the UHNM NHS Trust to institutionalise the change process as the data acquired informs the priority of the organisation. It allows the management to enhance the value for money through the assessment of demand and capacity metrics, which allow the Trust and the County Hospital to identify shirt in demand pressures, which also informs the distribution and allocation of healthcare resources. The County Hospital has institutionalised numerous changes such as the expansion of the outpatient facilities, particularly for the emergency access clinics, starting and refurbishing operating theatres and maternity units (UHNM 2017b). This is paramount as it incorporates the changes into the organisation through the institutionalisation of the transformation.

Leadership Approaches for Change Management

Transformational leaders are driven by the need to recognise and understand essential demands for change, which allows the modification of the existing environment to achieve ideal situations for supporting a successful transition (Van der Voet, 2014). This leads to the creation favourable population attitudes and control indications to monitor and address emerging issues and challenges throughout the transitioning process. Practical communication skills are paramount in transformational leadership due to the potential of inspiring confidence in people through administrative infrastructures (Ghasabeh et al., 2015). Notably, transformational leadership is applicable in different levels and fields of organisations and governance in the quest for the maximum possible efficiency. Current studies show that transformational leadership is made up four major components, including idealised influence, intellectual stimulation, individualised consideration, and inspirational motivation (Hayes, 2014). Nevertheless, communication stands out as a key customary requirement in significant leadership theories. This underscores the significance of including dialogue as an essential constituent in the assessment of transformational political leadership (Svendsen and Joensson, 2016). Besides, interaction process predominantly features as one of the most critical platforms for transformational leaders in politics.

Intellectual stimulation fosters the development of analytical and problem-solving skills. Transformative leaders inspire the followers in discovering innovative approaches in dealing with challenges hindering dream and vision actualisation (Doppelt, 2017). This improves quality products in decision-making organs and individual supporters. Intellectual stimulation facilitates the ability to solve widespread, recurring, and enduring problems using new techniques. High degrees of independence and autonomy are paramount in enhancing cognitive capabilities among the followers and leaders alike (Deschamps et al., 2016). Transformative political leaders can stimulate intellectual growth by championing the implementation of policies by investing in infrastructures and regulations supporting growth in education, science, research, art, and technology. These developments help in the identification of innovative analytical and problem-solving techniques. Advanced literacy potential is paramount in addressing typical challenges facing the society as it promotes inventive discoveries in resource utilisation and efficiency. Leaders must also lead by participating in activities supporting intellectual stimulation (Van der Voet, 2014). The resulting involvement boosts the followers' confidence in emulating their leaders.

Idealised influence compels transformational leaders to lead by examples. Charismatic personalities exhibited through internal and external morality inspires admirations, increasing the public confidence and trust in the leadership structures. Appealing qualities allow leaders to set moral standards, which reduces confrontational possibilities. Setting idealised moral values discourages the prevalence of corrupt dealings within the governing institutions, promoting efficient utilisation and distribution of public resources. Idealised influence inspires risk-taking initiatives to achieve social changes (Ghasabeh et al., 2015). Individualised considerations are paramount in addressing marginalisation since it promotes equity and equality in the distribution of opportunities, resources. It recognises unique needs, capabilities, and desires of the followers. Leaders are in a position to coach and nurture compassionate connections in which collaborative relationships are established (Deschamps et al., 2016). Appreciating individual contributions and potential boosts self-confidence, motivation, as well as energy replenishment among the followers. Individualised considerations also play an essential role in stimulating, nurturing, and coaching ambitious developments.

Inspirational motivation empowers transformational leaders to articulate explicit visions resonating with common social expectations and challenges. This amplifies the confidence and commitment among the followers, allowing a smooth introduction and implementation of transformative goals (Svendsen and Joensson, 2016). Inspiration traits provide a sense of purpose in pursuing transformational prosperity. Leaders with motivational and inspirational characteristics are often thorough, specific, engaging, comprehensive, influential and charming in describing or championing ambitious goals. Displaying relentless optimism and enthusiasm about the future encourages the followers to persevere and overcome obstacles between visionary expectations and shared experiences (Yang, 2016). Frequent communication fosters vigorous empowerment which is paramount in boosting the commitment of leaders and the followers towards achieving collective goals.

Transformational process require strong communication skills to actualise inspirational motivation, individualised considerations, intellectual stimulation, idealised influence and other qualities that make a good leader. Effective communication abilities are the most basic elements of socialisation and engagement (Gupta, 2011). An excellent communicator can trigger a debate that increases public awareness regarding available opportunities or areas in need of urgent address. Public discussions based on reliable facts gradually control social perceptions towards a predetermined direction. This allows the followers to consider critical matters in different perspectives increasing the potential of solving underlying problems (Pollack and Pollack, 2015). A leader can only inspire confidence in leadership structures and self-actualisation through rigid communication channels. Attaining self-confidence among the followers promotes the efficiency at which specific needs are identified and sufficiently addressed.

Justification and Conclusions

Change management is increasingly becoming paramount in the modern organisational environment. In this case, the organisational change at the Mid Staffordshire was triggered by major failure of in the care delivery. Increased number of deaths than projected was the major trigger that alerted the relevant authorities concerning the need to re-evaluate the entire management and make sustainable, feasible and practical recommendations, and eventually resolutions (Gupta, 2011). However, these changes require robust leadership structures, which enabled the transition management to the implementation of the final recommendations. Transformative leadership theory has been identified as one of the leading factor for effective change management (Pollack and Pollack, 2015). In this case, the five factors that are particularly significant for effective management and leadership of change are attributed to the five primary components of transformative leadership, namely, idealised influence, intellectual stimulation, individualised consideration, communication skills, and inspirational motivation.

Intellectual stimulation: The UHNM NHS Trust staff is continuously engaged in Health and Safety education along with Equality and Diversity training, which is fundamental in enhancing the quality of care delivered at the facility. The collaboration between the Stafford University and Keele University in learning, development, research and innovation stimulates the workforce to implement innovative ways to address the underlying problems facing the healthcare delivery process along with the institutions. Awareness campaigns especially concerning the significance of hygienic practices play a central role in enhancing the quality of services provided by the institutions. Besides, the contemporary staff continues to inspire the coming generation by guiding a new cohort of nurses, assistants, and midwives in attempts to stimulate intellectual development of the organisation (Manaseki-Holland et al., 2017).

Idealised influence: The County Hospital management has taken the initiative of participating in research and innovative research in collaboration with various learning institutions. This allows the management to influence the staffs in making sustained efforts that can improve the quality of treatment and the competence level. This has played a central role in transforming the hospital that was previously marred with chaotic services. Individualised consideration: The performance assessment is often done at different levels (UHNM, 2016). This is exemplified by the performance indicators at the team, committee, and Trust Board levels, which provides for data that can be used to enhance various aspects of the care delivery. Intensified training has enhanced the competence of the workforce to provide individualised care

(UHNM 2017b). Strong communications are visible in throughout the board as there are regular meetings with the board to update on the performance of various components of the hospital.

Briefly, change management is a process which requires extensive deliberations and planning, which can only be successful in the presence of robust leadership and management structures. Transformational leadership theories appear as the most convenient and effective model for change management. This is attributed to the fact that the model provides structured components that facilitate an effective change management process, ensuring that the transition is successfully handled and the last resolution is adopted accordingly. It ensures that sustainable measures are taken to ensure that the final goals are achieved by ensuring cumulative gains are observable and recognizable to those affected by the change.

References List

Bottle, A., Jarman, B. and Aylin, P., 2011. Strengths and weaknesses of hospital standardised mortality ratios. *BMj*, *342*, p.c7116.

Deschamps, C., Rinfret, N., Lagacé, M.C. and Privé, C., 2016. Transformational leadership and change: How leaders influence their followers' motivation through organizational justice. *Journal of Healthcare Management*, *61*(3), pp.194-213.

Dixon-Woods, M., Baker, R., Charles, K., Dawson, J., Jerzembek, G., Martin, G., McCarthy, I., McKee, L., Minion, J., Ozieranski, P. and Willars, J., 2013. Culture and behaviour in the English National Health Service: overview of lessons from a large multimethod study. *BMJ quality & safety*, pp.bmjqs-2013.

Doppelt, B., 2017. *Leading change toward sustainability: A change-management guide for business, government and civil society*. Routledge.

Francis, R., 2013. *Report of the Mid Staffordshire NHS Foundation Trust public inquiry: executive summary* (Vol. 947). The Stationery Office.

Ghasabeh, M.S., Soosay, C. and Reaiche, C., 2015. The emerging role of transformational leadership. *The Journal of Developing Areas*, *49*(6), pp.459-467.

Gupta, P., 2011. Leading innovation change-The Kotter way. *International Journal of Innovation Science*, *3*(3), pp.141-150.

Hayes, J., 2014. *The theory and practice of change management*. Palgrave Macmillan.

Kapur, N., 2014. Mid-Staffordshire hospital and the Francis report: what does psychology have to offer. *Psychologist*, *27*, pp.16-20.

Kotter, J.P. and Cohen, D., 2014. *Change Leadership: The Kotter Collection (5 Books)*. Harvard Business Review Press.

Mohammed, M.A., Lilford, R., Rudge, G., Holder, R. and Stevens, A., 2013. The findings of the Mid-Staffordshire Inquiry do not uphold the use of hospital standardized mortality ratios as a screening test for 'bad'hospitals. *QJM: An International Journal of Medicine*, *106*(9), pp.849-854.

Manaseki-Holland, S., Lilford, R.J., Bishop, J.R., Girling, A.J., Chen, Y.F., Chilton, P.J. and Hofer, T.P., 2017. Reviewing deaths in British and US hospitals: a study of two scales for assessing preventability. *BMJ Qual Saf*, *26*(5), pp.408-416.

Pollack, J. and Pollack, R., 2015. Using Kotter's eight stage process to manage an organisational change program: Presentation and practice. *Systemic Practice and Action Research*, *28*(1), pp.51-66.

Salge, T.O. and Schäfer, S., 2015. Failing to learn from failure. *Failure-driven innovation*. Berlin, Germany: artop.

Svendsen, M. and Joensson, T.S., 2016. Transformational leadership and change related voice behavior. *Leadership & Organization Development Journal*, *37*(3), pp.357-368.

Traynor, M., 2014. Caring after Francis: moral failure in nursing reconsidered. *Journal of Research in Nursing*, *19*(7-8), pp.546-556.

UHNM 2016. Annual Report 2014-2015 http://www.uhnm.nhs.uk/aboutus/Documents/AnnualReportsAndAccounts/Annual%20Report%202014-2015%20(FINAL).pdf

UHNM 2017a. Major Trauma Centre Ranked No.1 In The Country For Survival Rates http://www.uhnm.nhs.uk/news/Documents/UHNM%20News/UHNM%20News%20Issue%203.pdf

UHNM 2017b. Annual Report and Accounts For the year ended 31 March 2017 https://www.staffordshireandstokeontrent.nhs.uk/Annual%20Report/Annual%20Report%20and%20Accounts%202016-17.pdf

Van der Voet, J., 2014. The effectiveness and specificity of change management in a public organization: Transformational leadership and a bureaucratic organizational structure. *European Management Journal*, *32*(3), pp.373-382.

Yang, Y.F., 2016. Examining competing models of transformational leadership, leadership trust, change commitment, and job satisfaction. *Psychological reports*, *119*(1), pp.154-173.

YOUR KNOWLEDGE HAS VALUE

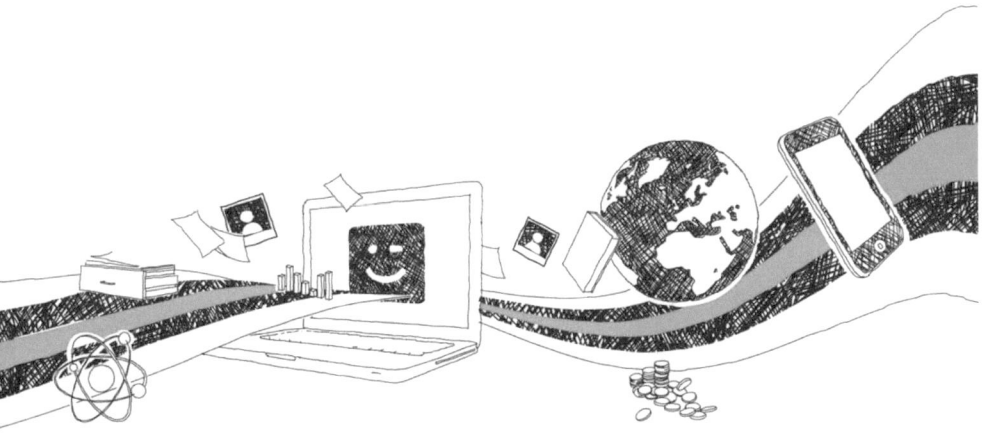

- We will publish your bachelor's and master's thesis, essays and papers

- Your own eBook and book - sold worldwide in all relevant shops

- Earn money with each sale

Upload your text at www.GRIN.com
and publish for free

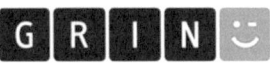